YOUR KNOWLEDGE HAS VALUE

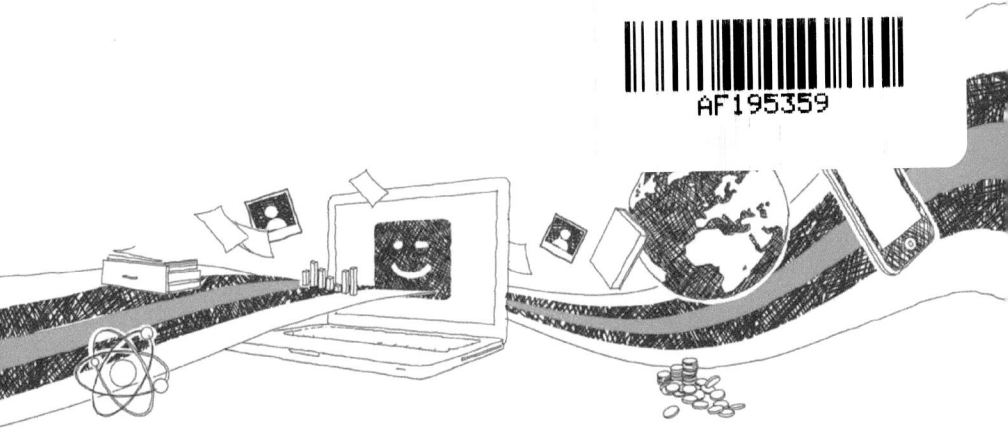

- We will publish your bachelor's and master's thesis, essays and papers

- Your own eBook and book -
  sold worldwide in all relevant shops

- Earn money with each sale

Upload your text at www.GRIN.com
and publish for free

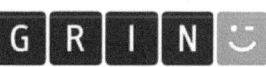

Joseph Manase, Enedy Mlaki

Conception of Vulnerability Forces to HIV/AIDS Infections among Secondary Schools Students in Tanzania

GRIN Publishing

Bibliographic information published by the German National Library:

The German National Library lists this publication in the National Bibliography; detailed bibliographic data are available on the Internet at http://dnb.dnb.de .

This book is copyright material and must not be copied, reproduced, transferred, distributed, leased, licensed or publicly performed or used in any way except as specifically permitted in writing by the publishers, as allowed under the terms and conditions under which it was purchased or as strictly permitted by applicable copyright law. Any unauthorized distribution or use of this text may be a direct infringement of the author s and publisher s rights and those responsible may be liable in law accordingly.

Imprint:

Copyright © 2012 GRIN Verlag, Open Publishing GmbH
Print and binding: Books on Demand GmbH, Norderstedt Germany
ISBN: 978-3-656-22222-4

This book at GRIN:

http://www.grin.com/en/e-book/195879/conception-of-vulnerability-forces-to-hiv-aids-infections-among-secondary

GRIN - Your knowledge has value

Since its foundation in 1998, GRIN has specialized in publishing academic texts by students, college teachers and other academics as e-book and printed book. The website www.grin.com is an ideal platform for presenting term papers, final papers, scientific essays, dissertations and specialist books.

Visit us on the internet:

http://www.grin.com/

http://www.facebook.com/grincom

http://www.twitter.com/grin_com

CONCEPTION OF VULNERABILITY FORCES TO HIV/AIDS INFECTIONS AMONG SECONDARY SCHOOLS STUDENTS IN TANZANIA

Joseph Manase & Enedy Mlaki

The University of Dodoma, College of Education, Department of Educational Foundations and Continuing Education(Community development Unit), P. O Box 523, Dodoma, Tanzania.

Abstract

The study designed to assess forces for vulnerability to HIV/AIDS infections among secondary schools students in Dodoma Municipality. Cross sectional survey was employed. Both probability and non probability techniques were used to obtain the sample. Objectives of the paper were to determine vulnerability forces to HIV/AIDS infection among students in Dodoma Municipal and identification of risk behaviors that lead to HIV/AIDS infection in the study location. Data analysis was done by statistical package for social science (SPSS) computer soft ware. The findings show that vulnerability forces leading to HIV/AIDS infection among students are among others, lack of awareness and drug abuse, High rate of HIV infection through blood transfusions and widespread sharing of contaminated injecting equipments were the risk forces for HIV/AIDS spread. Some media disseminates HIV/AIDS miss-information, prejudice and myth. Drug abuse, poverty, adolescence stage, peer group, ignorance, carelessness of the students and engagement in sexual intercourse were the main forces for HIV/AIDS spread. Finally it was recommended that Counseling agencies for HIV/AIDS to assist Peer group/friends, the community to fight against Female Genital Mutilations, agencies to disseminate HIV education to secondary students to increase their awareness. The government should empower the community economically for Poverty reduction. Integration of HIV/AIDS education in all social subjects curricula to be a must.

Key words: *vulnerability forces, HIV/AIDS, secondary school students, media, dissemination, education*

Introduction

Despite the world's third decade of the fight against HIV/ AIDS pandemic, the evidence of its impact is undeniably a profound human tragedy. It is a threat to the economies of the countries and of the resources and the capacities on which human security and development depends (UNAIDS, 2004). It is evident that HIV/AIDS pandemic is an increasing phenomenon in pa most parts of the world and needs somewhat combined efforts to mitigate this problem. Based on current information, about 33 million of the world population is living with the HIV virus, majority of whom are in their prime years as workers and parents. 45% of all new infections among adults are young people aged between 15-24 who are for this facts believed to be in their formal schools, more notably in secondary schools (UNAIDS, 2004).

Young people aged between 10-24 years are the AIDS generation, they have never known a world without AIDS of over 60 million people who have been infected with HIV/AIDS in past 20 years and about half of them become infected between the ages of 15-24 years. (URT, 1996). Over the 25 years of the AIDS epidemic in Tanzania, emphasis has been placed on the development of strategies and approaches to scale up the interventions and deal with the epidemic. Despite all the efforts that have been made the number of students infected continue to grow, students in urban areas have a higher prevalence in relations to those in rural areas (URT,2007).It is estimated that about 2.2 million people are living with the virus and about 400,000 are in need of anti-retroviral therapy. So it has been seen that the impact of the disease is almost incomprehensible. Consequences of the epidemic have been affecting all spheres of life (MOH, 2004).

The human resources loss has a serious social and economic impact in all sectors and at the community and individual levels. The flow of many opportunistic infections such as tuberculosis and some forms of cancer is a result of HIV infection. Increase in infections result in many resources being diverted from other areas to HIV prevention, care and treatment. Also it has been seen that poverty significantly influences the spread of HIV/AIDS, which ultimately leads to a loss of the most productive segment of the society, leading to reduction of income and suffering for individuals and communities.students on the other hand are in a group that is being infected in an alarming rate in Dodoma Municipality (MoEVT,2008).This paper in particular seeks to find out key vulnerability factors leading to HIV/AIDS infection among secondary school students in Dodoma, Tanzania.

Students are a group which is vulnerable to HIV/AIDS and other STDs in Tanzania and Dodoma in particular. The knowledge of teenage students, boys and girls is lower than that of their older ones due to the fact that there is an increase in HIV infections for teenage students in the region. Kapinga (1991) reported that students were less likely to be informed from the mass media than the grown up people due to the Tanzania social-cultural context, although the results of the study did not confirm this.

The government of Tanzania through various agencies has been educating young people, especially students to avoid AIDS infections by being involved in various life styles. The impact of this education is seen to bring no significant improvement in terms of lessening HIV infections among students in Dodoma. There is, instead, an increase in HIV infections among students in the country, Dodoma Municipality in particular. This study therefore, intends to assess factors leading to students' vulnerability to HIV/AIDS in Dodoma Municipality.

This study intended to determine the vulnerability factors to HIV/AIDS infection among students in Dodoma Municipal, identify risk behaviors that lead to HIV/AIDS infection, identify the sources of HIV/AIDS information for students and identify the factors leading to HIV/AIDS transmission in Dodoma Municipality.

Reviewed Literature

Vulnerability of HIV/AIDS among Students at Global Level

AIDS Is considered as one of the most devastating stating public health problems in recent history. In June 2000, the centers for Diseases control and prevention (CDC) reported that 120,223 (includes only those cases in areas that have confidential HIV reporting). Since the beginning of the HIV/AIDS epidemic about 65 million people have been infected with HIV and 28 million people have died of AIDS. In 2003, an estimated 40 million people worldwide were living with HIV, five million of who were newly infected. More than three million people died of AIDS in 2003. The most at risk of HIV/AIDS are young people. About 6,000 people aged between 15 and 24 get infected with HIV every day (Heelen, 1990).

Globally, between 5 and 10 percent of all HIV infections result from injecting drugs but in some countries it is more than 50 percent. Injecting drug uses (IDUs) are a key population group to target to prevent the spread of HIV/AIDS. Unfortunately, in most countries, the response has been grossly inadequate and has had little impact upon HIV rates among IDUs. Some countries, however, have managed to prevent, slow or stop the spread of HIV/AIDS among IDUs. They have achieved this by adopting wide ranging harm reduction programs (Heguye, 1995).

In the late 1970s HIV entered the United States. By then shooting galleries, places where people buy, prepare and inject drugs, were fully established. In this setting, widespread sharing of contaminated injecting equipment occurred and HIV spread rapidly. Since the start of the epidemic, 36 percent of all AIDS cases have been directly, or indirectly, linked to injecting drug use. Over half of all women infected with HIV in the United States are either drug users of the sexual partners of drug user (Berlin, 1990).

Most children who are born with infections of HIV have one or other parent who is a drug user. Needle and Syringe Programs (NSPs) are now found in 39 of the 50 states but most programs are too small to reach the estimated 1 – 1.5 million IDUs. Some cities, such as New York, have seen a reduction in HIV incidence among IDUs attending NSPs but overall the United States has failed to cope with the dual HIV/AIDS epidemic (WHO, 1995).

The government structures of the Soviet Union, Eastern Europe and Central Asia collapsed in the late 1980's and early 1990's following years of economic crisis and social unrest. Many people sought escape from the hardship and growing social uncertainties and turned to drugs. At the same time the illicit drug industry flourished (Lugoe, 1996). A rapid spread of drug injecting reached epidemic proportions and this new phenomenon coincided with an explosive HIV/AIDS epidemic. An estimated four million IDUs live in the region and an estimated 1.2 million people in the region have HIV/AIDS. Injecting drugs is the primary mode of transmission: in Russia drug use. Currently only 11 percent of IDUs in the region have access to harm reduction programs.

In the United States there are HIV positive, and 311,701 are living with AIDS. Of these patients, 44% are gay or bisexual men, 20% are heterosexual intravenous drug users, and 17% are women. In addition, approximately 1000-2000 children are born each year with HIV infection. The world Health Organization (WHO) estimates that 33million adults and 1.3 million children worldwide were living with HIV/AIDS in 1999 with 5.4 million being newly infected that year. Most of these cases are in the developing countries of Asia and Africa.

Vulnerable Populations at Greatest Risk
Country data indicate that the number of people living with HIV continues to rise in all parts of the world despite the fact that effective prevention strategies exist. Sub-Saharan Africa remains the hardest-hit region with extremely high HIV prevalence among pregnant women

aged 15-24 reported in a number of countries. In Asia, for example the HIV epidemic remains largely concentrated in injecting drug users, men who have sex with men, sex workers, clients of sex workers and their immediate sexual partners. Effective prevention programming coverage in these populations is adequate. Diverse epidemics are under way in Eastern Europe and Central Asia. Injecting drug use is the main driving force behind epidemics across the region (Kenya, 1995).

In many high-income countries, sex between men plays an important role in the epidemic. Drug injecting plays a varying role. In 2002, it accounted for more than 10% of all reported HIV infections in Western Europe and was responsible for 25% of HIV infections in North America.

In Latin America and the Caribbean, 11 countries have an estimated national HIV prevalence of 1% or more (WHO, 1995).

In Sub-Sahara Africa, heterosexual transmission is by far the predominant mode of HIV transmission. Unsafe injections in health-care settings are believed to be responsible for around 2.5% of all infections. Recently, it has been suggested that unsafe medical injections account for most HIV transmission in the region (Gisselquist *et al.*, 2002). However, a recent thorough review of the evidence concluded that, while a serious issue, unsafe injections are not common enough to play a dominant role in HIV transmission in Sub-Saharan Africa (Schmid, 2004).

The 'unsafe injections' theory does not take into account the possibility that people sick of HIV-related disease might receive more injections. Moreover, the pattern of injections in health-care settings does not match sub-Saharan Africa's HIV-infection distribution pattern by age and sex. Although the safety of injections must be assured in all health-care settings, effective strategies addressing sexual transmission have the largest potential to turn the epidemic around in this region (Sawaya et al.,1995).

Vulnerability to HIV/AIDS among Students National Level

Ministry of Health (MOH, 1996) estimated that the number of AIDS cases was around 400,000 at the end of 1995. Furthermore, the numbers of HIV-infected people and AIDS cases in the year 2000 are anticipated to reach million and 2.4 million, respectively (MOH, 1995). Lugoe (1996) reported that 1.6% of the male cases and 6.0% of the female cases of a total of 31,247 AIDS cases reported to the MOH between 1987 and 1994 occurred in persons aged 15-19, and that 8.5% of the male and 21.5% of the female cases occurred in those aged 20-25. WHO (1995) warned that up to two third of new HIV infection in many of the developing countries may be occurring in 15 to 24 years old and up to 60% of infection in females may be occurring by the age of 20. Adolescents in Tanzania are thus at great risk of HIV infection (Hunter, 1991).

Sexual transmission of HIV can be prevented by using condoms during sexual relationships, assuming that they are used correctly and consistently. Although condoms are available in Tanzania, there are many constraints on their use by Tanzanian adolescents. Many religious leaders and elders see use of condom as a message promoting adolescent sexual activity, and the Tanzanian government has therefore not effectively emphasized the promotion of condom use among adolescents (World Bank, 1992; Talle, 1995). There is no official AIDS in Tanzania education programmes in the school curriculum and previous studies in Tanzania have shown that condom use is not popular enough to effectively prevent HIV infection (Kapinga *et al.,* 1991; Sawaya *et al.,* 1995).

Very little information, however, has been documented concerning the influence on HIV-risky adolescent, sexual behaviour of attitudes and opinions on condom use, as well as AIDS-related knowledge, information sources, risk perception and attitudes. The Risk-1group consists of students who are sexually active and do not always use condoms. The Risk-2 group is the portion of the Risk-1 group who has had multiple sexual partners in the past year. The Risk-2 group, therefore, has higher risk of infection than the rest of the Risk-1 group (Pattullo 1994). Most students get information on AIDS through mass media and through communication with friends, parents, teachers, religious leaders and health personnel. This is an encouraging finding in terms of continuing the promotion of AIDS education through radio, newspaper, and television and personal/group communication.

Personal communications generally encouraging in the absence of a formal AIDS education programmed in the school curriculum, but such communication may also be a source of mis-information, prejudice and myth (Lule and Gruer, 1991: Pattullo *et al.,* 1994). In the recent study, those getting information from friends were engaging in Risk behavior more than others, and there is a need to find out what quality of information is being passed through communication with friends. Introduction of proper AIDS education in the school curriculum minimize misconception sand prejudice, and encourage communication with parents. Involving people who are living with HIV/AIDS in school AIDS education, as successfully done in developed countries (Carballo *et al.,* 1995; Sapa-AP, 1996), would be helpful for students to more deeply understand people who are living with HIV/AIDS.

However, the knowledge of teenage students and girls is lower than that of the older ones and boys (Kapiga *et al.,* 1991) reported that girls were less likely to be informed from the mass media than boys due to the Tanzanian socio-cultural context, although the results of the present study did not confirm this. Introducing AIDS education in the lower grades of schools and paying special attention to girls being effective. Students with good knowledge concerning HIV transmission tended to engage in Risk-1 behaviour. Those taking Risk-1 and/or Risk -2 behaviour appear to generally understand that they are at high risk of getting HIV infection. About half of the students feel that condoms are not safe and that condoms can bring disease, and two-thirds feel that condoms reduce the sensation of romantic sex (Heguye, 1995).

Many young bar workers in northern Tanzania believe that condoms are HIV infested and expressed fear of using them (Talle et al., 1995). Partner's anti-condom bias associated with both Risk-1 and Risk-2 behaviors. In both cases, better information and education on condoms through proper sources would reduce anti-condom bias. Such bias can only be effectively modified if the government promotes condoms in a much more active way (Lule and Gruer, 1991). There is therefore a need to educate these students that the risk of HIV infection exists in a personal sense and the need to protect them is very important. Alcohol drinking associated with Risk- behaviour should also be considered in future AIDS educational programmes. Drinking alcohol, smoking cigarettes and attending disco are positively associated with sexual activities in northern Tanzania (Lugoe et al., 1995).

Adolescents in Massachusetts who drink alcohol and use drugs were less likely to use condoms (Hingson et al., 1990). Health education in schools should therefore provide particular focus on those who are engaging in such behavior. One-quarter of the students thought that they were at risk of HIV infection and they were more likely to engage in risk. Those who were prepared to test their HIV status were less likely to engage in Risk behaviour.

The results of the present study suggest that there are two kinds of students with respect to AIDS risk. Students of one group are not involved in risky sex and relatively free from HIV infection. Students of the other group are involved in risky sex, though they are aware both of their risk and the usefulness of condoms for AIDS prevention. They are receiving misconceptions from their friends and tending to strongly dislike condom use, as well as drinking alcohol and fearing to take the HIV test. The contents and methods of health education for these two groups should be different. For the fist group, the purpose is to prevent them from being involved in risky sex by giving accurate knowledge on concerning romantic love, HIV infection and AIDS, and safe sex. Health educators could impart knowledge on a variety of safe-subtopics, teaching students that there are other, safe ways for gaining the pleasure of romantic love.

For the latter group who were already involved in risky sex, information disseminated through the mass media and mass education may not be sufficient to change their attitudes and behaviour. Education aimed at giving more knowledge would seem to be of least use for them, and their education should be focused more on changing their behaviour and attitudes. Condom use may be more effectively promoted by means of face-to-face discussions and focus group discussion in school programmers.HIV tests, counseling based on the results of the tests and follow up small group discussion/learning with health education specialists may be effective. The social norms prohibiting sexual activities among adolescents seemed to be less effective than previously.

These norms are less influential because of modernization processes (religion, education, economy, culture, politics, etc.). In much of Tanzanian societies, the teaching of sexual knowledge and skills to young people is regarded as immoral as a result, children grow to adolescence and into young adulthood without being given any systematic training in these matters (Heguye, 1995).

Strategies to Reduce HIV Transmission

HIV/AIDS has become a national barrier towards development (URT, 2007). To combat such obstacle encouraged initiation of several strategies, among them being the establishment of the National policy on HIV/AIDS. This policy gives several objectives and one of them is the prevention of the transmission of HIV/AIDS. Attention being on multiple sexual partners in order to enable to adopt safer sex practices (URT, 2001).

The second issue is to consider community involvement as that help to consider community involvement as that help to curb the HIV/AIDS epidemic. The third is gender issue in relation to HIV/AIDS specifically gender equity and promotion of equal participation of man and women for negotiating safer sexual practices and empowering women to say NO to Unsafe sex (URT, 2001). That prevention can be done at individual when they change their behaviour against HIV/AIDS particularly through education awareness and information on HIV/AIDS. The forth issue is to consider community involvement as that help to curb the HIV/AIDS epidemic. The third is gender issue in relation to HIV/AIDS specifically gender equity and promotion of equal participation of man and women for negotiating safer sexual practices and empowering women to say NO to Unsafe sex (URT, 2001). That prevention can be done at individual when they change their behaviour against HIV/AIDS particularly through education awareness and information on HIV/AIDS.

Methods

The study employed cross sectional survey design where data were collected at one point in time by means of questionnaire and interview schedule. Both quantitative and qualitative research paradigms were employed and simple random and purposeful samplings were used to select shools and students respectively. Schools which were selected, are Kiwanja cha ndege, Nkuhungu , Miyuji ,Dodoma and Viwandani secondary Schools. These are the schools which are located at the centre of Dodoma town and their students are said to face a great deal of HIV infection challenges. Total of 31 secondary school students responded to the questionnaire and only 9 students from Dodoma secondary were used in a focused group discussion.

Students who were involved are form 2, 3, and 4, Inclusion criteria of these forms are because they have knowledge and experience about school life. And exclusion criteria for form 1 students are due to the lack of experience and knowledge about school life. Quantitative data were analyzed using statistical package for Social Sciences (SPSS) version 17, to determine frequencies, percentages and mean of the corresponding statements.

Results of the Study

This section presents the findings of the data analysis of the study together with their interpretations. Forty (40) students were used to provide information related to the study.31 questionnaires were subjected to SPSS for analysis. Presentation of the findings is in descriptive statics. Presentation of the results is organized according to the research questions investigated. The presentation is done by use of tables and figures where necessary. The tables for data are presented in frequencies and percentages while tables showing data according to research questions are presented in frequencies, percentages, mean and rank ordering in order to minimize the span of the data during discussion.

School analysis

The respondents were asked to indicate their school. The findings were as categorized in table 1 below:

Table 1: Study area (N=31)

Schools	Frequency	Percent
Miyuji	8	25.8
Nkuhungu	7	22.6
K/ndege	8	25.8
Viwandani	8	25.8
Total	**31**	**100.0**

From table 1 above, it is evident that majority of the respondents are equal who are Viwandani and K/Ndege secondary schools(25.8%) as compared to the Miyuji (25.8%)and Nkuhungu (22.6%)

Sex analysis

The respondents were asked to indicate their sex. The findings were categorized in table 2 below

Table 2: (N=31) Frequency and Percentage distribution of Respondents according to sex

Sex		Frequency	Percent
Valid	Male	15	48.4
	Female	16	51.6
	Total	**31**	**100.0**

The results from table 2 above shows that majority of the respondents were females (51.6%) as compared to the males (48.4%).However, the difference is seen to be too marginal.

Age analysis

Table 3: (N=31) Age range of the Respondents

	Age range	Frequency	Percent
Valid	13-16	14	45.2
	17-20	15	48.4
	24-27	01	3.2
	5.00	01	3.2
	Total	31	100.0

The findings from the above table show that majority of the respondents are those who ranged between 17-20 years (48.4%).It is between teenage and early adulthood and therefore are at a high risk.

Analysis of who take care of the student

There were four categories of respondents. These are single, both parents, step father, guardians.

Frequency distribution of the respondents according to the guardians of the respondents.

Table 4:. Study areas (N=31)

	Category of guardian	Frequency	Percent
Valid	Single	07	22.6
	Both parents	17	54.8
	Step father	01	3.2
	Guardian	06	19.4
	Total	31	100.0

Majority of the respondents were cared by their both parents 17(54.8%) followed by those who lived with single parent 7(22.6%) and the ones who cared by guardians 6(19%).From the analysis it can be presented that about 45.2% of the students are not cared by both parents,this implies that some of the forces to HIV/AIDS can act upon them since they are not cared by both parents and hence vulnerable to those factors.

Research question one; what are the vulnerability factors to HIV/AIDS infection among students in Dodoma Municipality?

Table 5: Determination of the vulnerability factors to HIV/AIDS infection in Dodoma Municipality.

No	Item	Reponses									
		5		4		3		2		1	
		N	%	N	%	N	%	N	%	N	%	Mean
1	I insist that poverty is the factor for HIV vulnerability among students.	19	61.3	10	32.3	1	3.2	0	0	1	3.2	3.7
2	Peer groups (friends) can be a reason for being vulnerable to HIV/AIDS	13	41.9	12	38.7	2	6.5	2	6.5	2	6.5	3.5
3	Distance from Home to school is the factor of being vulnerable to HIV/AIDS.	6	19.4	16	51.6	7	22.6	1	3.2	1	3.2	2.194
4	Raping is reason for HIV/AIDS vulnerability among secondary school students.	14	45.2	10	32.3	4	12.9	2	6.5	1	3.2	1.9032
5	I believe that students-teachers relationship is a factor for HIV vulnerability.	9	29.0	12	38.7	4	12.9	3	9.7	3	9.7	4
6	Drug abuse and addiction is the reason for students vulnerability to HIV/AIDS	16	51.6	8	25.8	3	9.7	1	3.2	3	9.7	4.1
7	Female genital mutilation is the factor for vulnerability to HIV/AIDS among secondary school students.	17	54.8	6	19.4	3	9.7	3	9.7	2	6.5	3.00
8	Care for HIV victims is a factor of vulnerability HIV/AIDS among students.	5	16.1	4	12.9	4	12.9	2	6.5	16	51.6	3.65
9	Early Age at sexual initiation is a factor of vulnerability for HIV/AIDS.	17	54.8	5	16.1	3	9.7	3	9.7	3	9.7	4.00

| 10 | Lack of awareness is a factor of vulnerability of HIV/AIDS among students. | 11 | 35.5 | 15 | 48.4 | 3 | 9.7 | 0 | 0 | 2 | 6.5 | 1.94 |

Results from table 5 above shows that majority (7 responses) of the respondents agrees with the truth that the mentioned factors are the reasons for the students vulnerability to HIV infection in Dodoma Municipality. some of the statements fell under the disagree category, none of the statements fell under the strongly agree, not sure status or strongly disagree. It is also seen that, majority of the respondents are convinced with the factors mentioned above. However on ranking, the highest factor had a mean of 4.1 while the lowest scored 1.90.

Research questions two; What are the risk behaviors that lead HIV/AIDS?

Table 6: Determination of the risk behaviors that lead to HIV/AIDS infection.

No	Item	Reponses										
		5		4		3		2		1		
		N	%	N	%	N	%	N	%	N	%	Mean
1	I believe that engaging in unprotected sex is the cause of HIV/AIDS transmission.	16	51.6	13	41.9	2	6.5	0	0	0	0	1.54
2	I believe that sharing of the sharp things like injection, Lazar blade, needles, combs are the causes of HIV/AIDS transmission.	9	29.0	12	38.7	4	12.9	3	9.7	3	9.7	4.00
3	Kissing (Wet kiss) is believed to be a factor of HIV/AIDS transmission.	19	61.3	3	9.7	5	16.1	0	0	4	12.9	4.00
4	Dry kissing is believed to be a factor of HIV/AIDS transmission.	2	6.5	2	6.5	6	19.4	5	16.1	16	51.6	1.93
5	Sharing of clothes is among the factor of HIV/AIDS transmission among students.	5	16.1	2	6.5	5	16.1	5	16.1	14	45.2	3.68
6	Blood transfusion spread AIDS among students	15	48.4	4	12.9	2	6.5	2	6.5	8	25.8	2.48

| 7 | Sharing food with infected victims. | 1 | 3.2 | 2 | 6.5 | 2 | 6.5 | 2 | 6.5 | 24 | 77.4 | 4.48 |
| 8 | I believe that playing together is the factor of transmitting HIV/AIDS. | 16 | 51.6 | 8 | 25.8 | 3 | 9.7 | 1 | 3.2 | 3 | 9.7 | 4.1 |

Results from table 6 above shows that majority of the respondents agrees with the fact that the mentioned factors are key factors for the transmission of HIV/AIDS among students in Dodoma municipality. Few statements indicate negative response.

. However on ranking the highest factor had a mean of 4.48 while the lowest factor scored equal mean of 1.54.

Discussion

Research question one: What are the vulnerability factors leading to HIV/AIDS infection among secondary school students in Dodoma Municipality?

The tabulated information in table 5 indicates that, majority of the respondents agreed on the factors that lead to the vulnerability to HIV/AIDS infections among secondary school students as Drug abuse and addiction, Lack of awareness on HIV/AIDS prevention and other predetermined factors.

The present findings are in line with Kenya (1995) whose study revealed that injecting drug use is the main driving force behind epidemics across the region. The findings do not conquer with Hingson et al.,(1990) who argues that adolescents who drink alcohol and use drugs were less likely to use condoms and hence encountered a threat of being infected by HIV. However the findings also are in line with (Lugoe et al., 1995) who argues drinking alcohol, smoking cigarettes and attending disco positively associated with sexual activities. Health education in the school curriculum would minimize the misconceptions about HIV/AIDS Infection.

The study findings indicated also that vulnerability to HIV/AIDS among students is due to lack of awareness on HIV/AIDS prevention. The findings are in line with (Carballo *et al.,* 1995; Sapa-AP, 1996) whose study recommends involving people who are living with HIV/AIDS in school AIDS education, would be helpful for students to more deeply understand people who are living with HIV/AIDS.

Researcher findings about the knowledge indicate that introduction of proper HIV/AIDS education in the school curriculum would minimize the misconceptions about HIV/AIDS infection and this finding is in congruence with the study by Carballo et al., (1995, 1996) who contends that, if HIV/AIDS education is introduced in the school curriculum, it would lessen to a great extent the likelihood of infections among students in primary and secondary schools.

The present study of researchers shows that prevention of HIV/AIDS can be done at individual when they change their behavior against HIV/AIDS particularly through education awareness and information on HIV/AIDS. Also gender issue in relation to HIV/AIDS specifically gender equity and promotion of equal participation of man and women for negotiating. Safer sexual practices and empowering women to say no to unsafe sex (URT, 2001).

Research questions two; what are the risk behaviours that lead to HIV/AIDS infections?
Information tabulated in table 6 indicate that majority of respondents were aware of risk behaviours that lead to HIV/AIDS infections as ranked on the table. The findings are in line with Gisselquist *et al.,* (2002) who argues that unsafe medical injections during blood transfusion account for most HIV transmission. The findings are also supported by the study by (Othiambo, 1994) which revealed high rate of HIV infection through blood transfusions

due to widespread sharing of contaminated injecting equipment like syringes, needles, and razor blades and other sharp metallic objects.

Through focused group discussion, students were asked on the sources through which they get information about HIV/AIDS. The findings reveal that most students get information about HIV/AIDS through mass media and through communication with friends, parents, teachers, religious leaders and health personnel probably due to reliable sources that are available to them. This implies that students had access of information regarding HIV/AIDS and it contradicts with the notion of most parents and educators perceptions that students lack the most important education about HIV/AIDS. This is an encouraging finding in terms of continuing the promotion of AIDS education through radio, newspaper, and television and persona/group communication. Despite of the available media communication the researcher sees some communication as a source of mis-information, prejudice and myth, this is on line with Lule and Gruer, (1991) and Pattullo *et al.,* (1994) whose study revealed that those getting information from friends were engaging in Risk behaviuor more than others.

Similarly the researchers' views on miss-information about HIV/AIDS prevention is in conjunction with the study by Heguye (1995) who argues that the teaching of sexual knowledge and skills to young people is regarded as an immoral as a result, children grow to adolescence and into young adulthood without being given any systematic training in these matters with a focus to Tanzania context. It follows therefore that there is a need to find out what quality of information is being passed through communication with friends and through which media. This is again supported with a study by Lule and Gruer, (1991) which convey that, in both cases, better information and education on condoms through proper sources would reduce anti-condom bias. Such bias can only be effectively modified if the government promotes condoms in a much more active way.

Conclusions and Recommendations

The study was designed to assess the forces for vulnerability to HIV/AIDS infections among secondary schools students in Dodoma Municipality in Tanzania. The study was extended to determine the vulnerability factors to HIV/AIDS infection among students in Dodoma Municipality, identifying risk behaviours that lead to HIV/AIDS infection, and identifying the sources of HIV/AIDS information for students. The findings showed that;

vulnerability factors lead to HIV/AIDS infection among secondary school students in Dodoma Municipality include among others, lack of enough risk awareness and drug abuse, high rate of HIV infection through blood transfusions and widespread sharing of contaminated injecting equipments are the risk forces for HIV/AIDS spread. Some media communication disseminates HIV/AIDS miss-information, prejudice and myth, drug abuse, poverty, adolescence stage, peer group, ignorance; careless of the students and engagement in sexual intercourse are the main factors for HIV/AIDS spread in Dodoma Municipality.

Recommendations

Based on the specific objectives it is recommended that;

Counseling agencies for HIV/AIDS to assist Peer group/friends, the community to fight against Female Genital Mutilations (FGM), the agencies for HIV/AIDS to disseminate HIV education to secondary students to increase their awareness. The agencies empower for health and Red Cross society to take care on blood transfusion, the government to the community economically for Poverty reduction, the ministry of education and vocational training to include in curriculum the HIV/AIDS education programme. It is also recommended that, religious institutions to play role on provide religious ethics to the members of community, agencies for the media information to effectively and efficiently disseminate HIV/AIDS education through Television, radio, internet and Newspapers.

REFERENCES

Carballo, M/and Kenya, P. I. (1995) Behavioral issues and AIDS. Essex,

Drucker E. (1999). Drug Prohibition and Public Health: 25 years of Evidence. Public Health Report. January/February Vol 114: pp14-29.

Heguye, E. S. (1995). Young people's perception of sexuality and condom use in Kahe.

K. I., Biswalo, P. M.and Talle, A. (1995) *Young People at Risk: Fighting AIDS in Northern Tanzania.* Scandinavian University Press, Oslo, pp. 107-120.

Kapiga, S. H., Nachtigal, G. and Hunter, D. J. (1991) Knowledge of AIDS among secondary school pupils in Bagamoyo and Dar-es-Salaam, Tanzania. *AIDS,* **5, 325**-328.

Lugoe, W. L. (1996) Prediction of Tanzanian Students HIV Risk and Prevention Behavior. University of Bergen, Norway.

Lugoe, W. L., Klepp, K. L, Rise, J., Skutle, A. and Biswalo,P. M. (1995) Relationship between sexual experience and non-sexual behaviours among secondary school students in Arusha, Tanzania. East African Medical Journal, 72,635-640.

Lule, G. S. and Gruer, L. D. (1991) Sexual behaviour and use of the condom among Ugandan students. AIDS Care, 3, 11-19.Ministry of Health, Tanzania (1995) National Policy on HIV/AIDS/STD. National AIDS Control Programme, Version 3.

Mboup, S., Kanki, P. J. and Kalengayi,M. R. (eds) (1994). AIDS in Africa. Raven Press, New York, pp. 497-511 .Hingson.

K., Moses, S. and Plummer, F.A. (1994) . Survey of knowledge, behavior and attitudes relating to HIV infection and AIDS among Kenyan secondary school students. AIDS Care, 6, 173-181.

R. W., Strunin, L., Berlin, B. M. and Heelen, T.(1990) Beliefs about AIDS, use of alcohol and drugs, and unprotected sex among Massachusetts adolescents American Journal of Public Health, 80, 295-299.

Sawaya, M., Fimbo, B., Owenya, F. and Mkoba, S. (1995) Tanzania HIV/AIDS/STD education in schools.

Sapa-AP (1996). AIDS-Johnson. Magic Johnson brings AIDS awareness campaign for Soweto, Johannesburg.

Talle, A. (1995). Bar workers at the border.TACAIDS, Dar es Salaam.

The World Bank (1992) A World Bank Countiy Study: Tanzanian AIDS Assessments and Planning study. World Bank, Washington, DC, pp. 149-151.

WHO (1990) Research Package: Knowledge, Attitudes, Beliefs and Practices on AIDS (KABP). Phase 1. WHO, Geneva.